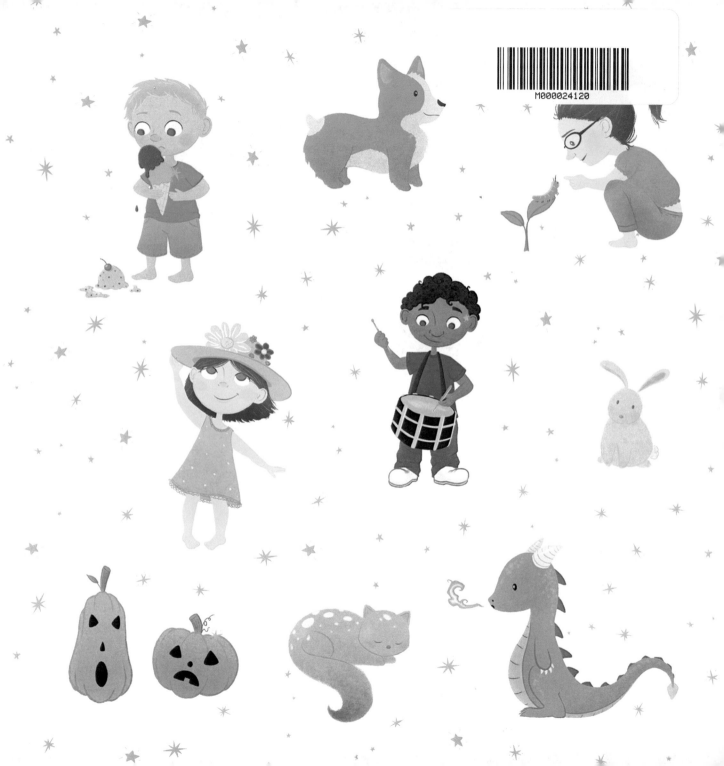

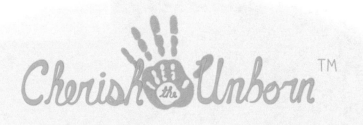

Hello in THERE!

POETRY TO READ TO THE UNBORN BABY

WRITTEN by: Carole Marsh Longmeyer
illustRATED by: Allie Conzola

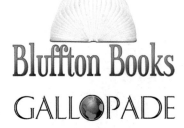

Bluffton Books

GALLOPADE

MOTHER is the name for God
in the lips and hearts of children.
—William Makepeace Thackeray: VANITY FAIR

Where did you come from, baby dear?
Out of the everywhere into here.
—George Macdonald: AT THE BACK OF THE NORTH WIND

Copyright 2015
Carole Marsh Longmeyer

For rights, permissions, quotations, comments, and more,
you can reach the author at carole@gallopade.com

Illustrations by Allie Conzola
Book design by Susan Van Denhende
Art Director John Hanson

Through Love to Light by Richard W. Gilder (1849-1909)

COMPANION

Cherish the Unborn™

BOOK:

Nine Months in My Mommy: Autobiography of an Unborn Baby

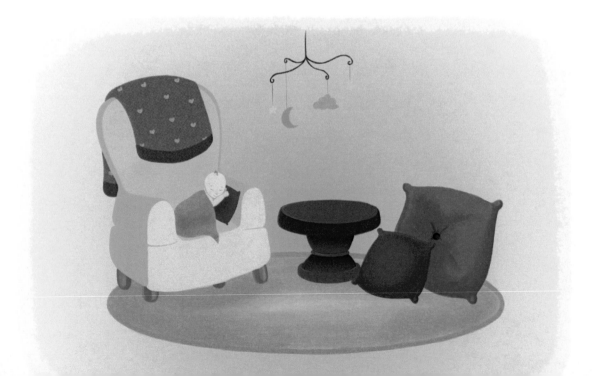

Lullaby
to the
Unborn

Child in chamber
Sleeping nigh,
Hear this muffled
Lullaby.

Song to keep you
Company;
Until I'm with you,
And you're
With me.

The dreams
You dream,
Are preparation,
For the time
Of your
Creation.

Nativity,
Nativity,
Sleep and be,
Sleep and be

Infant curling
In my womb,
Know that there is
Endless room,
In my life and
In my heart.
Never, never shall we part,
Even at the time of birth
Even at the time of birth
Celebration!
Celebration!!

Little one
From God you came,
Precious baby
Is your name
All will never
Be the same.

When you come
When you come

Lullaby of love,
An echo
Hearts that beat
Until you let go,
Drummers go
From two to one,
Different drummers,
Share one drum
Until you come
Until you come
Celebration!
Celebration!
Nativity
Nativity
Sleep and be
Sleep and be

✳ ✳ ✳

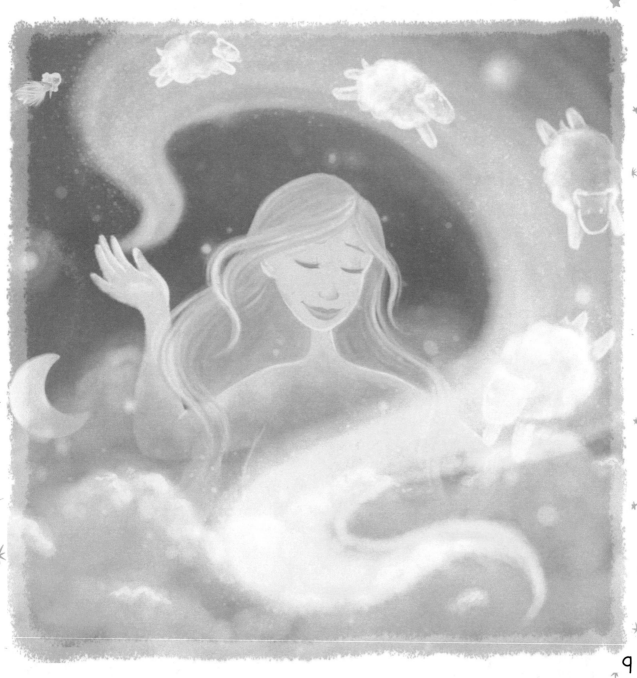

Before I Was . . .

Before I was, I was . . .

Star Dust
Seashell Crumbs
Sunbeam Bits
Teddy Bear Fuzz
Lightning Flash Flakes
Moonlight Mist
Foxfire Flames
Dew Droplets
Smoke Curls
An Angel's Shadow
Baby's Breath
Wave Wisps
Rainbow Seeds

What was you?

✳ ✴ ✳

Rainbow Butter

Baby, oh Baby,
Wait until you see
All the colors
There will be!

Purple is one you're sure to adore,
It's black plus blue plus something more;
It's everything from antique lavender lace
To the grape jam and jelly
You'll smear on your face!

Gold and silver are special hues,
They're holiday colors,
(And birthday, too!)
Sunshine and moonlight,
Honey and stars,
Diamonds and fireflies,
And fast-moving cars!

Black is a color
You'll see with me,
Outside at night,
Behind the tree.
(But we'll curl cozy in your nursery!)

Brown is the color of gingerbread;
It may even be the color of the hair on your head!
Chocolate's brown, and a teddy bear friend,
And the color of pudding you'll love to play in!

Blue is the color of sky and sea;
Even the color your eyes may be;
Blue is the color grandma's bring,
In surprise-baby packages tied up with string!

There's a funny color known as gray,
The color of squirrels and mice at play;
Pussy willows and nanny goats,
And the waves that bob
Under little toy boats.

White will be a favorite for you,
The color of milk, snow, lace and sand,
Book pages, ice cream, flowers, and . . .
The pure, true love of
Your Mom and Dad.

Orange is a color
You'll love to see,
On a snowman's nose,
Or an autumn tree.

I wonder what you'll
Think of pink?
A stuffed pink bunny
You'll love, I think!
(I think, in fact —
You'll be
Tickled pink!)
Pink's also the color of the tip of your thumb,
And, oh-my-goodness—bubblegum!

And, oh, there's green,
The color of grass,
A birthday balloon,
Limeade in a glass,
Grasshoppers, pickles,
And peppermint,
And the color of Spring
The sunshine sent!

Yellow's a color that's lots of fun,
From a fuzzy, little duckling,
To a lemon-stuffed bun;
Daffodils and dandelions,
Candlelight and daisies,
And the warm toasty glow
That will give us the lazies,
When we sprawl beneath
The summer sun awhile;
And golden yellow's the color
Of baby's smile!

Red will be your favorite color,
Your ball, your wagon,
A blanket you lay on,
To watch red fireworks up above,
And Valentine hearts are the color of love.
Red is a ride on grandpa's knee,
The color of the circus, the zoo, and the sound of
"Wheeeeee!"

We'll polish the colors and keep them bright,
Baby, oh, baby—won't you love your first sight!

* ✳ ✳

Baby's ABCs

A is for the awful day
When you'll grow up and go away.
(See how much I miss you so,
And you're not even here yet and have no place to go!)

B is for a boy,
If that is what you be,
(Even unborn, _you_ know—
But not yet me!)

C is for your first cry—
I can't wait to hear it, and I don't know why!
It's bound to be a joyful
"WHAAIIIIIIIIIIIIIIIIIIIIIIIIIII!"

D is for the drama
Of the day that you appear;
Don't be surprised to see me cry,
Or Dad to give a cheer!

E is for the evenings
When you'll snuggle into bed,
Lamplight like a halo
Will fall upon your head.

F is for the family fun
We'll count on.
But there's no rush—we'll give you time
To grow and come along!

G is for the goodness
Growing in your heart,
And a bond between us,
That never will depart.

H is for your happiness,
I wish for with all my heart.
May you with love be always blessed,
And Cupid find your heart!

I is for invisible
(That's what you'll hope that I
Think you are when we play
The game of old "Peep-Eye!")

17

J is for the jack-o-lantern
We'll carve when you are two:
"BOO!"
"BOO!"

K is for the balls you'll
Kick, kick, kick!
Or slap around
With a hockey stick!

L is for love
And lots and lots of it!
And Valentine candy
You'll eat in a bit.

M is for meander,
Through the park we will.
Down through a green forest,
And up a happy hill.

N is for the word "No!"
(You might as well start learning it now!)
We'll get through the Terrible Twos and potty-training,
But right now, I'm not sure how!

O is for the openness of your
Mind, heart and life.
And the joy of a wedding to
Husband or wife.

P is for persnickety;
A good kind of picky you will be,
To choose the things you want for yourself,
From a big red Harley to an Elf on the Shelf.

Q is for quick, quick, quick!
You'll want to see and taste and try it all—
Now, now, now!
Go on—have a ball!

R is for roly-poly baby games
You'll play on your belly and back,
With friends you don't have yet, but will,
With names like Jenny and Jack.

S is for serendipity—
The surprises you'll uncover!
The quirky paths life can take,
With so many joys to discover.

T is for treasures:
Experiences and memories,
Gold doubloons and the knees of bees,
And even carrots and fresh green peas!

U is for unicorns and other tall tales
We'll read together,
Creating memories
To last forever.

V is for voracious—
Your appetite for food and life and love!
And knowing you'll achieve your heart's desires
With guidance from God above.

W is for windows to the world:
Look! See!
Wow! Gee!
Go to Mars? You'll give it a whirl!

X is for eXceptional:
You'll be so, I guarantee.
At whatever you do, and besides,
I'll support whatever you'll be.

Y is for you, you, you,
And me, me, me,
And the family that
We soon will be!

Z is for the zzzzzzzz sounds you'll make,
Soft snoring as you sleep,
You'll look so precious in your crib,
That I'm sure that I will weep!

* * *

Nom de (Bebe) Plume

What shall we name you, baby?
How shall we call you near?
Elegant? Cutsey-pie? Faddish?
Or after Uncle Van der Veer?
I'll read a few from this list, dear,
Kick when you like one you hear!

Adrienne or Akaba?
Andersen or Yoyoma?

Boris? Doris? Morris? Duke?
Jose? Babette? Babar? Luke?

Caldecot or Carigiet?
Canby? Charlip? or Remay?

Diska? Em? Fatio? Fischer? Flora?
Francois? Hogogrian? Ivan? Ledora?

Mordrinoff? Munari?
Newberry? Nicholson?

Perrault or Piatti?
Rojankowsky or Ransom?

Seignobosc or Stephan?
Sugitar or Stobbs?

Titus? Ubrey? Ungerer?
Welber? Weise? Wahab?

Xavier? Yashima? or Zimnick?
Xena? Yettima? or Zo?

I haven't felt a foot yet, dear—
So how about Anna or Joe?!

✷ ✹ ✸

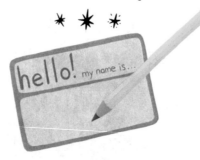

Babybet

A is a long-legged ladder

B is a big-bellied babysitter

C is a crescent moon

D is a drawer pull for your dresser

E is a shelf for your diapers and onesies

F is a rack for hanging your clothes

G is a waiter who serves up your food

H is the bed that you'll get when you grow

24

I is a kid you may know

J is his best friend

K is a kicker of balls

L waits . . . very straight

M is a map showing this way and that

N is a Z fallen over

O is a mouth that wants feeding

P is B's top-heavy sister

Q is a hoop and a stick

25

R is ready to run to the store

S is the way that she gets there

T is the table we'll eat on

U is the home of unborns

V is the bottom of a Valentine's heart, or the tip-end of your candy corn

W is a baby's bottom

X marks the stuff you're not to touch!

Y is a twig waiting to bloom

Z is the sound of you sleeping.

* ✳ ✳

Hello in there!

Hello in there!
Can you hear me?

Here's the sunshine—
Can you see?

I'm eating pizza—
Can you taste
The rich and sweet
Tomato paste?

I sniff a rose
Down to your well,
And wonder if
Its scent you smell?

With my palm
Upon my skin,
Can you feel
The warmth within?

27

I can't wait
Until you are here,
And find out all
The answers, dear!

* * *

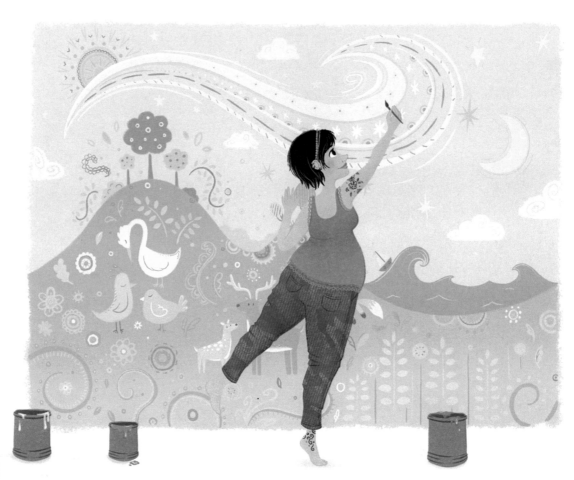

Rewriting the World

While I've been waiting
For your entrance,
I've been busy,
You might say.

The world was fine
For me and dad,
But before you come,
I thought I had

Better see to a few changes;
You might call them "rearranges" —
And so, I'm working hard and fast,
To sew up a peace that lasts.

I told Mother Nature
I thought it best
She lay volcanoes
Down to rest.

And while at it,
Tell tornadoes
To calm down and
Grow tomatoes!

And the wild-hair hurricanes
To make thunder and lightning friends.

Next, I told the distant lands
That you can't swim—
So, please hold hands.

"Fire?" I begged, "don't be too hot..
Snow—don't be so cold."
Days and years—
Let there be lots,
But time should
Not grow old.

Planets and stars
Should hold their place,
The moon put on
A happy face.

30

And just like any
Good brother or sister,
I've asked the birds
And bees to whisper.

Endless tiny details,
I think I've covered all,
Now, even if the bough breaks—
The cradle won't fall!

* * *

The Facts of Life

Before on your birth journey you go,
There are some things that you should know:

Life—it is not always fair,
About some things it will not care.

Bodies are made of mostly dust,
They do grow old and sometimes rust,

Love's not always easily found,
Often, you must search around,

Fears and tears are part and parcel
Of some days which will be a hassle,

Death is birth—but in reverse,
It's not something you rehearse.

But the fact is, as you know:
Life's the only way to go!

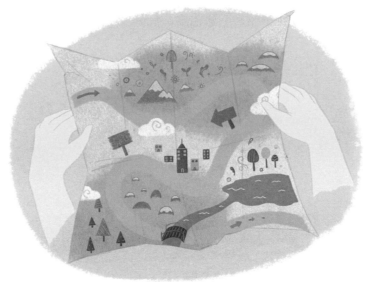

Surprise Store

We're saving lots of surprises
Outside here for you,
The list is almost endless,
So I'll just name a few:

Christmas morn

Candy corn

Kitty cats

Flowered hats

Puppy dogs

Crackling logs

Rain

Spain

Down escalators

Up elevators

Ice cream licks

Magic tricks

Sand pails

Fairy tales

Wiggling
Giggling
Red wagons
Blue dragons
Big hugs
Small bugs
Snowflakes
Cupcakes
Beaches
Peaches
Seashells
Jingle bells
Talking
Walking
Jet planes
Fast trains
Clowns
Towns
Toy boats
Billy goats

Rhinos

Dinos

Cars

Stars

Drums

Plums

Bananas

Pianos

Sun

Fun

Rhymes

Limes

Laughs

Baths

Old Tunes

New Moons

Bunnies

"Funnies"

Jack-O-Lanterns

Planet Saturn

35

Moms
Dads
Stripes
Plaids
Popcorn
Being born!

* * *

Birth

A grand and majestic entrance
Onto the stage of life
Celebrity, already,
Applause and "Bravo!"
Greet thee,
Friends and family
Meet thee:
Take a bow!

A world-class sunrise
Bursting forth
In beauty,
Glaring light, the bright
Dawn of a new
Beginning, new and
Welcome

Attainment of the mountain peak,
Discovery, journey,
Push on, push on,
Destination,
Victory

A wisdom, knowledge,
Understanding, comprehension,
Knowing, perception,
Perfect, yet
If not,
It does not matter

Promises fulfilled,
Destiny fulfilled,
Cosmic evolution,
Plan unfolding,
Life unfurling,
Colors whirling,
Circle curling,
Birth!

* * *

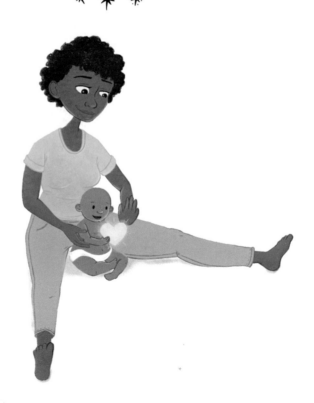

Through Love

Through love to light,
Oh, wonderful the way,
That leads from darkness,
To this perfect day!

From darkness,
And from sorrow of the night
To morning that
Comes singing o'er the sea

Through love to light,
Through light, oh, life,
To thee!
Oh, love, of love,
The eternal
Light
Of
Life

✱ ✻ ✳

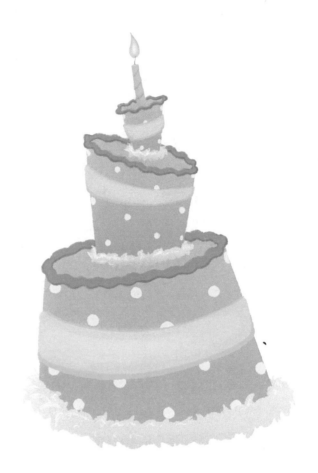

Happy Birthday!

Happy birthday to you!
Happy birthday to you!
Happy birthday, newborn baby,
Happy birthday to you!

Welcome to the world!
Welcome to the world!
Our welcome, newborn baby,
We're glad to see you!

How old are you?
How old are you?
How old, birthday baby,
How old are you?

I'm nine months old!
I'm nine months old!
Happy birthday to me!
I'm nine months old!

And glad to see you!
And glad to see you!
I knew you were there somewhere!
I'm glad to see you!

* * *

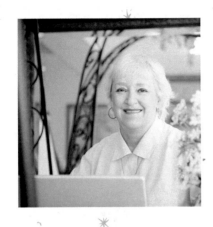

Carole Marsh was born 3 months early ("So I could be a Capricorn!") and weighed 1lb and 8oz. She could fit in the palm of her father's hand. Nurses fed her with an eye-dropper. She went home after 3 months in the Kennesaw Military Hospital, outside of Atlanta. For more than 30 years, she has written fiction and non-fiction for children ages 7-14. The author lives in coastal South Carolina with her husband.

Allie Conzola is an illustrator from Savannah, Georgia. She currently attends the Savannah College of Art and Design. She has a passion for creating characters and telling stories. When she is not drawing, she loves exploring nature, watching movies, and drinking large amounts of coffee! To view more of her work, visit be.net/allie-conzola.

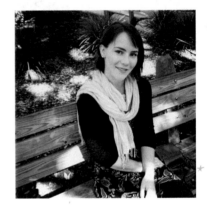

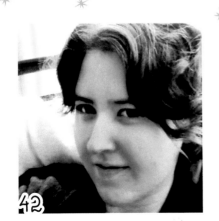

Susan Van Denhende was born with a really long last name that most people find hard to pronounce. It wasn't until middle school that she discovered she'd also been born with a talent and passion for art. Since then, she has graduated from the Savannah College of Art and Design and is now happily working to bring stories to children of all ages. You can find her work at be.net/auroradesilva.

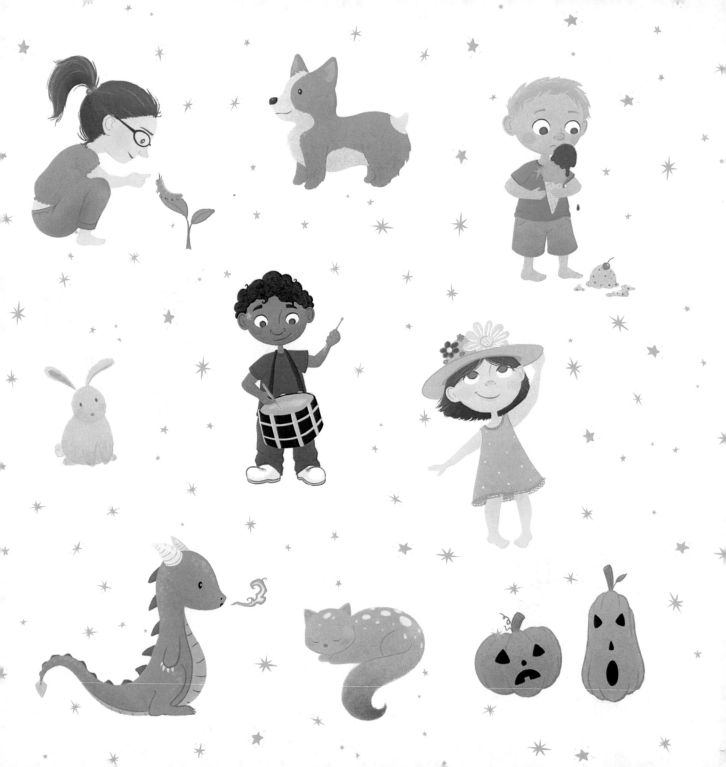